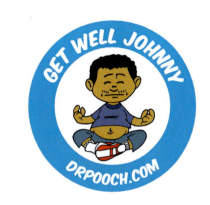

GET WELL JOHNNY
Book 5: Allergy Season!

By Dr. Pooch

Illustrations by Cuzzin' Dave

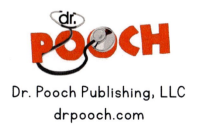

Dr. Pooch Publishing, LLC
drpooch.com

Get Well Johnny
Book 5: Allergy Season!
Copyright © 2015 by Dr. Pooch
Published by Dr. Pooch Publishing, LLC

ALL RIGHTS RESERVED. No part of this book shall be reproduced without written consent from the publisher, except for brief excerpts for the purpose of review.

DISCLAIMER: Dr. Pooch is NOT a medical doctor. Therefore, the information within this book is for educational purposes only. It should not be used as a substitute for professional medical advice, diagnosis or treatment regarding your or your child's well-being.

ISBN: 978-0-9964667-4-5

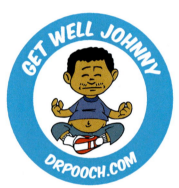

The Dr. Pooch Foundation

The Dr. Pooch Foundation is a nonprofit 501(c)(3) organization whose mission is to create and implement holistic health curriculum for schools and communities across the world. To change our world, we must begin with ourselves. Dr. Pooch Foundation programs increase and cultivate health and wellness awareness and nurture holistic health literacy. We are all connected to the whole. Let's learn new healthy ways and unlearn old destructive habits together to make a better more sustainable world for us ALL!

Donations and contributions to the Dr. Pooch Foundation go a long way towards increasing resources to ensure every child is not only health-literate, but holistic health-literate! Scan this QR Code to DONATE!

For more info: visit **drpooch.com**

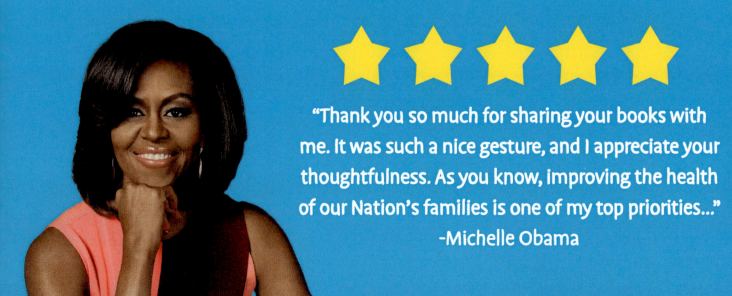

"Thank you so much for sharing your books with me. It was such a nice gesture, and I appreciate your thoughtfulness. As you know, improving the health of our Nation's families is one of my top priorities..."
-Michelle Obama

ACKNOWLEDGMENTS

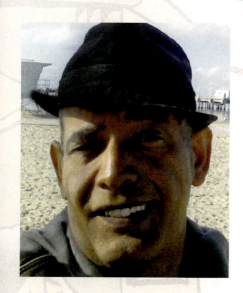

This book is dedicated to Dave "Cuzzin' Dave" Rodriguez, who lost his battle with cancer during the making of this book series. He was a one-of-a-kind guy with a great sense of humanity and humor.

Before the "Get Well Johnny" series, Cuzzin' Dave worked on Charlie Brown, Teenage Mutant Ninja Turtles and more. May his memory be honored by any who've gained insight from the wisdom within this book.
May you rest in peace, Cuzzin' Dave.

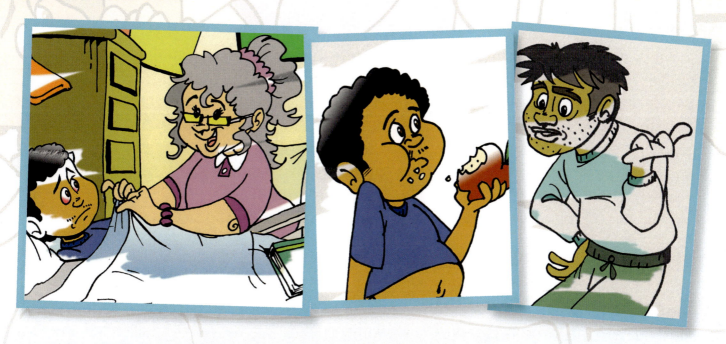

SPECIAL THANKS

The Dr. Pooch Foundation would like to acknowledge and give special thanks to the incredible creative team behind the **Get Well Johnny Book Series.** *This has been an incredible creative journey. The Dr. Pooch Foundation, Parents, Educators, and the Children of the world thank you from the bottom of our hearts.*

- **STORIES:** Writer Dr. Pooch, Hassan Diop (drpooch.com)
- **PHOTOGRAPHY:** Many photos by Weyni Hussien (work4weyni@gmail.com)
- **BOOK DESIGN AND EDITING:** Graphic Designer Alida Verduzco (alidaverduzco.com)
- **COVER DESIGN:** Artist Robel Fikremariam (robel79@gmail.com)
- **BOOK ILLUSTRATION (Books 7-12):** Illustrator Ilinda Pennant (ilinda.pennant@gmail.com) brought to life the pencil sketches that Cuzzin' Dave left unfinished.

NOTE TO PARENTS

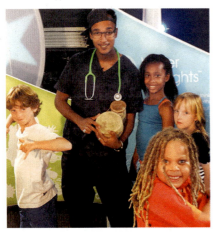

Allergic conditions have been increasing at alarming rates in our modernized world of synthetics and toxins. According to the Asthma and Allergy Foundation of America, allergies are the most common conditions affecting children. These terrible, persistent health problems are the 6th leading cause of chronic illness in the U.S.

Allergies, by definition, are when our bodies form antibodies against certain allergens. These allergens could be from pets, fabrics, dust mites, pollen, air pollutants, etc. However, the conversation about allergic conditions should also evolve to include the association of parasitic infections. Yes, PARASITES! Young people with parasitic worms may have an increased risk for allergies and asthma. Parasites may also be associated with behavioral issues, cardiomyopathy, delayed cognitive development, and impaired nutrition.

Increasingly, food allergies have become more and more frequent all over the world. Many studies have explored the environmental and nutritional changes that contribute to how people react to foods as well as the appearance of new food allergies. Whether as a response to parasites, modified food proteins, or environmental factors, the way our bodies react to modern foods has evolved. The introduction of hybridized (genetically modified) wheat, for example, has increased the gluten content of this grain 500-fold from what our foremothers and forefathers ate! No wonder gluten intolerances and allergies are occurring so frequently. Gluten (a glue-like substance) and casein (the sticky milk protein used to make glue... Ever notice the cow on Elmer's glue!?) may increase sensitivity in people already infected with parasites.

Parasitic infections are more common than you would think. For example, according to the Centers for Disease Control and Prevention (CDC), about 5% of the U.S. population has antibodies to the Toxocara parasite (roundworm), suggesting that tens of millions of Americans may be exposed yearly. That is just one of many thousands of existing parasites. Veterinarians recommend that you de-worm your pets every three months. Yet, how many times have you and/or your child been cleansed of parasites? If you or your child has Allergies, Leaky Gut Syndrome, Chronic Illness or Fatigue, Eczema, Psoriasis, Autism and more... you may want to find an adequate de-worming method. Natural periodic herbal cleanses including foods and medicines such as wormwood, cloves, black walnut and even sweet fruits such as dates are great at eliminating these unwanted guests for good!

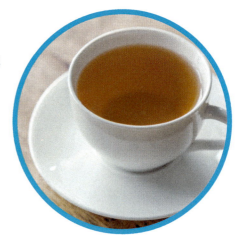

THANK YOU FOR YOUR DEDICATION TO A HEALTHY FUTURE!
-Dr. Pooch

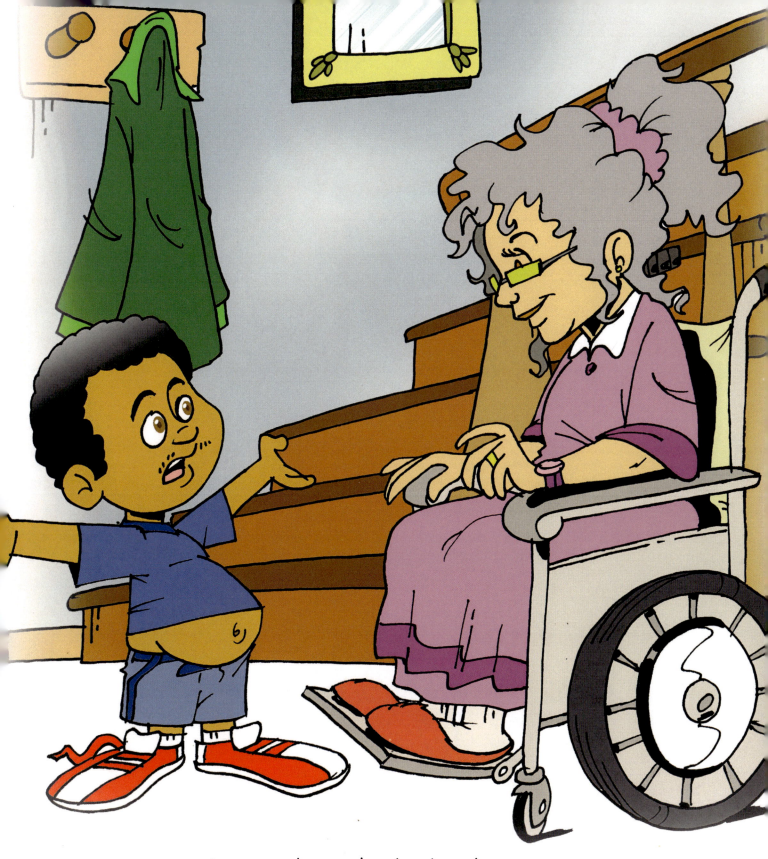

Mustache asked Abuela to
read a story before bed one night.
Abuela said, "Go to sleep, Johnny Mustache,
and don't let the bed bugs bite."

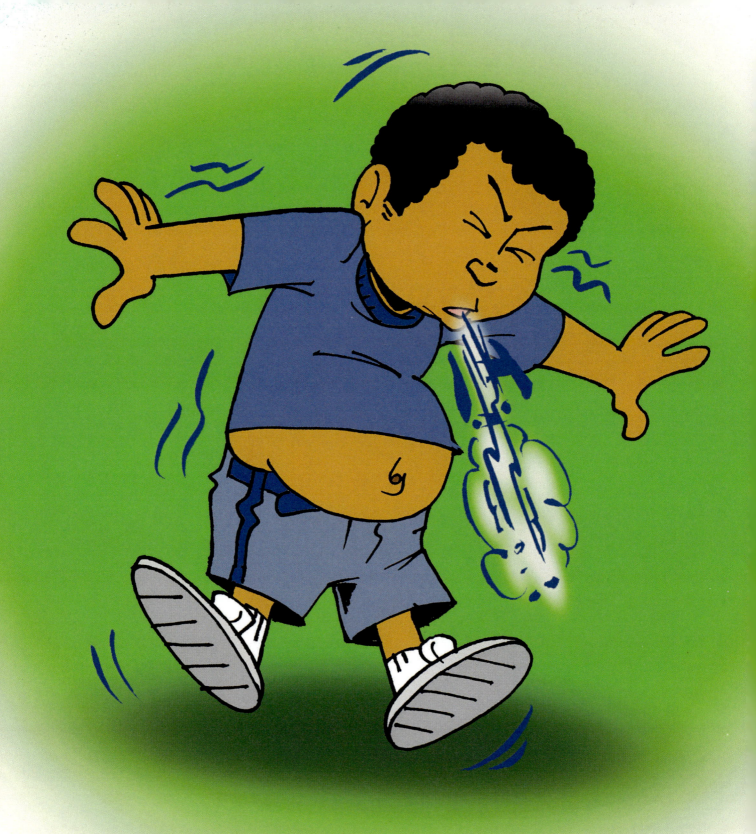

He replied with pleas
and, just then, he sneezed!
She said, "Bless you, my love,"
then decided to read.

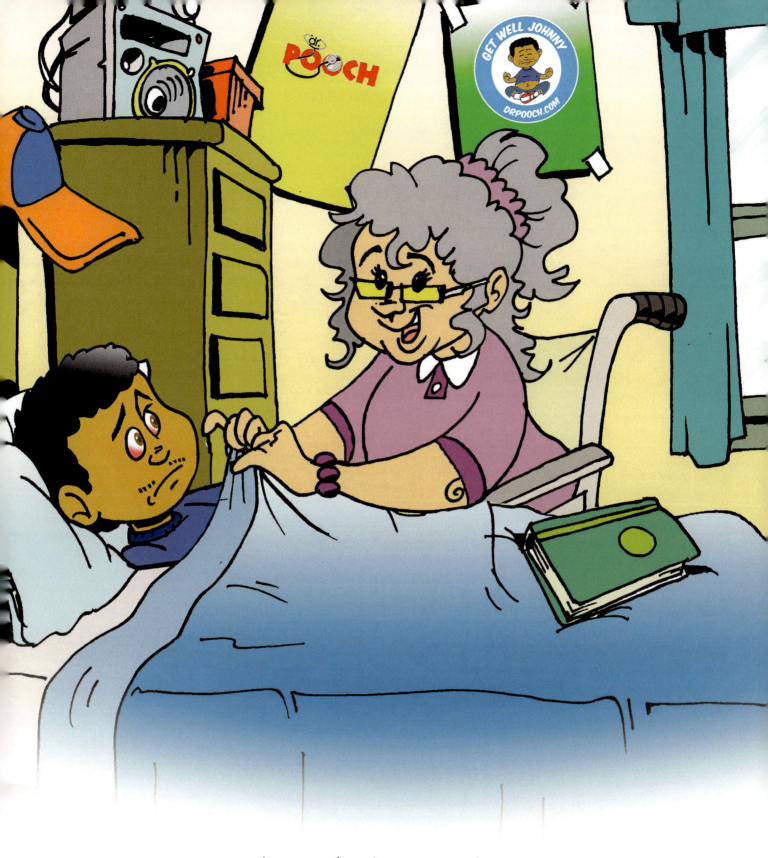

She tucked Mustache under covers and sheets, and said, "This is the story of a man with allergies..."

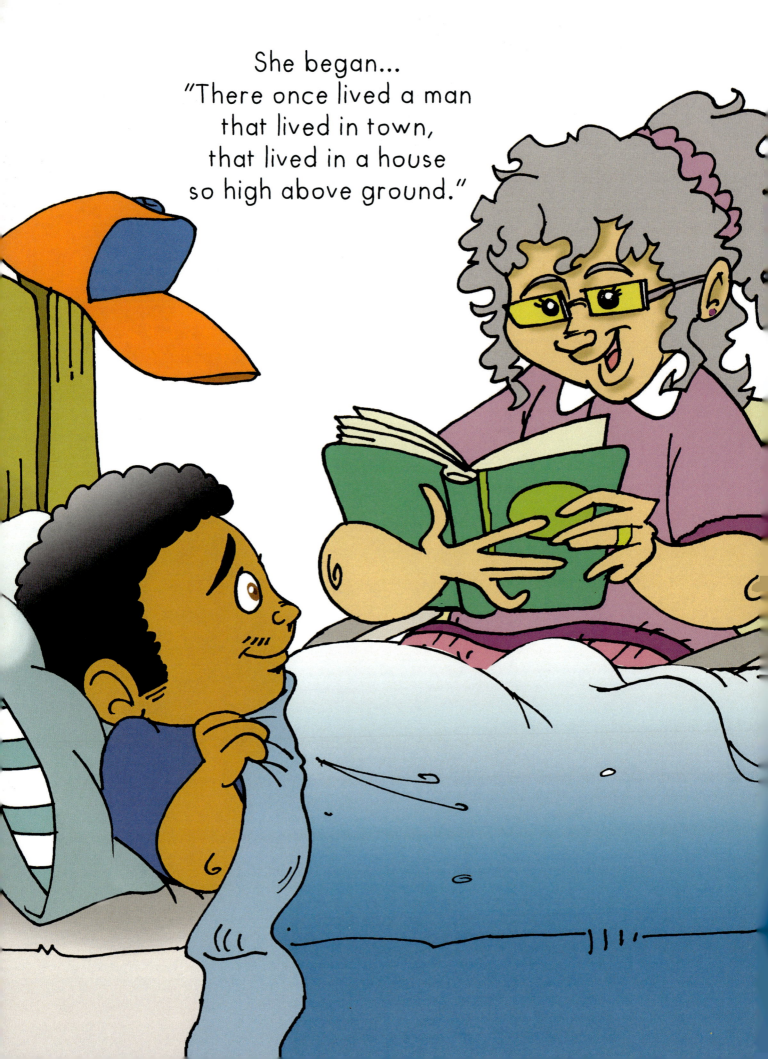

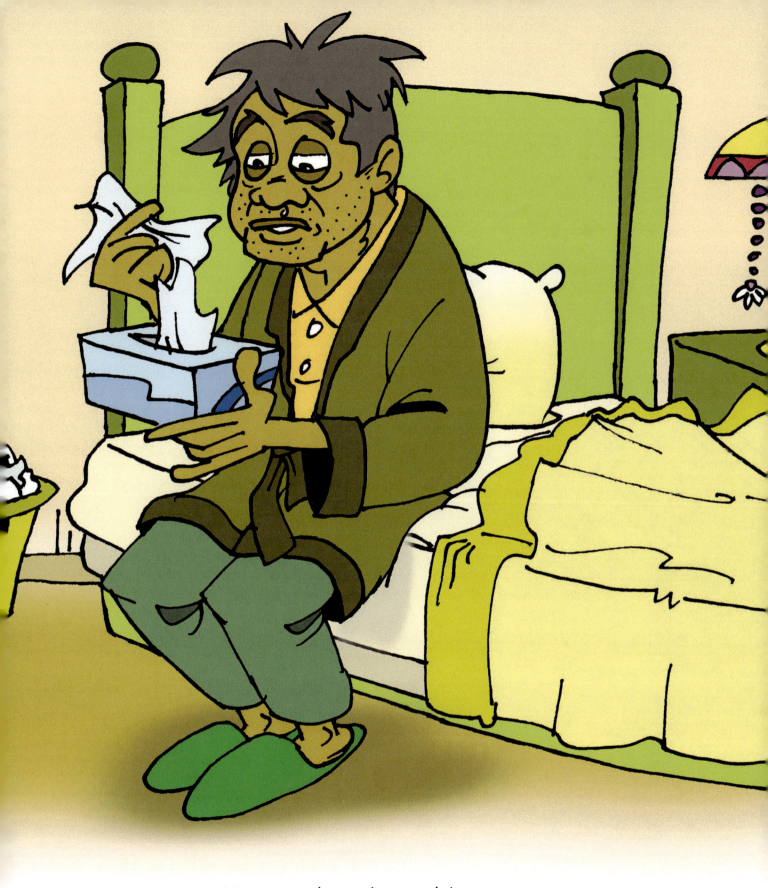

He cried and would weep
for days and for weeks.
Coughing and sneezing,
he barely could sleep.

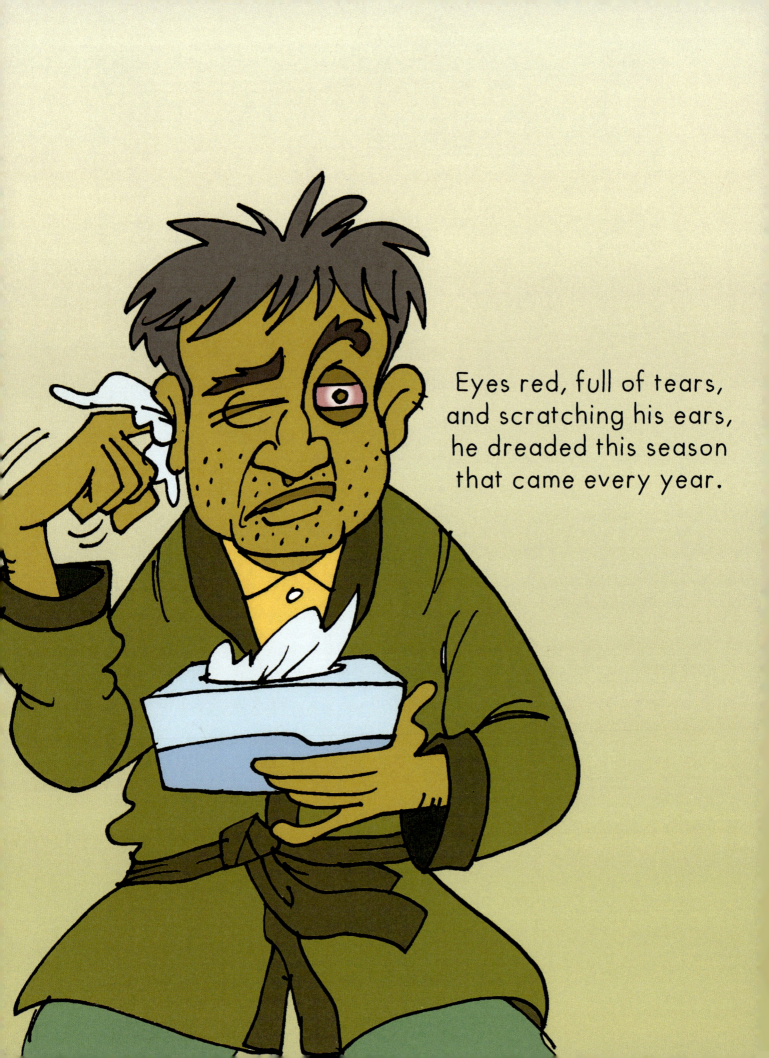

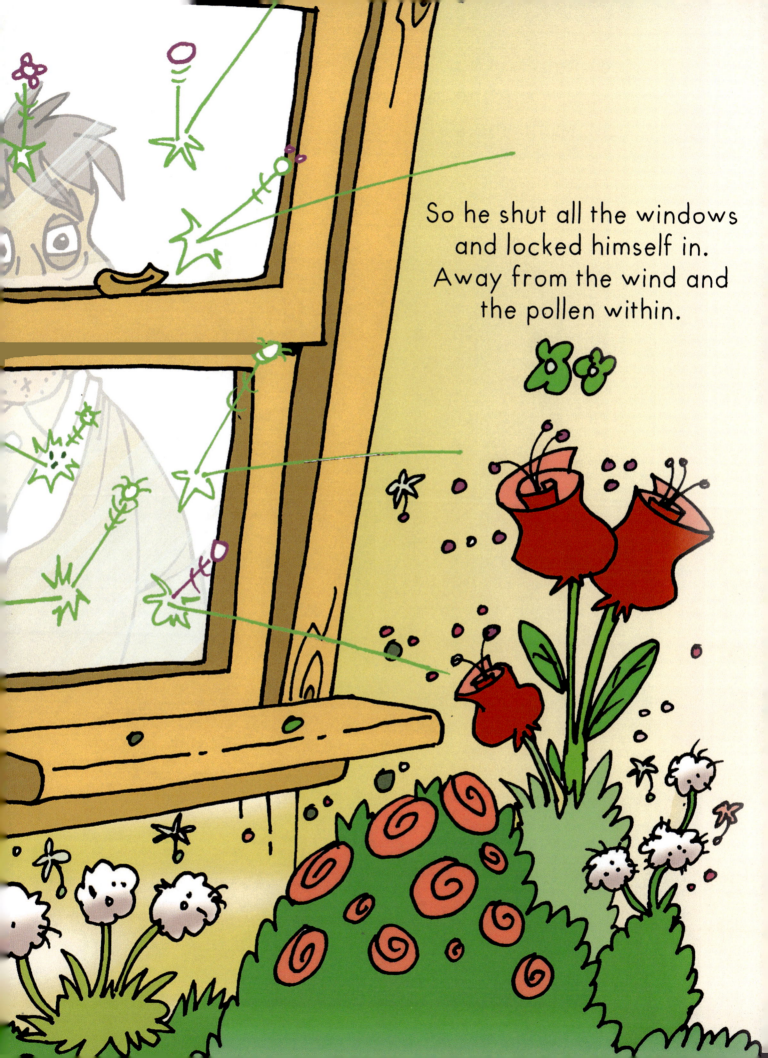

So he shut all the windows and locked himself in. Away from the wind and the pollen within.

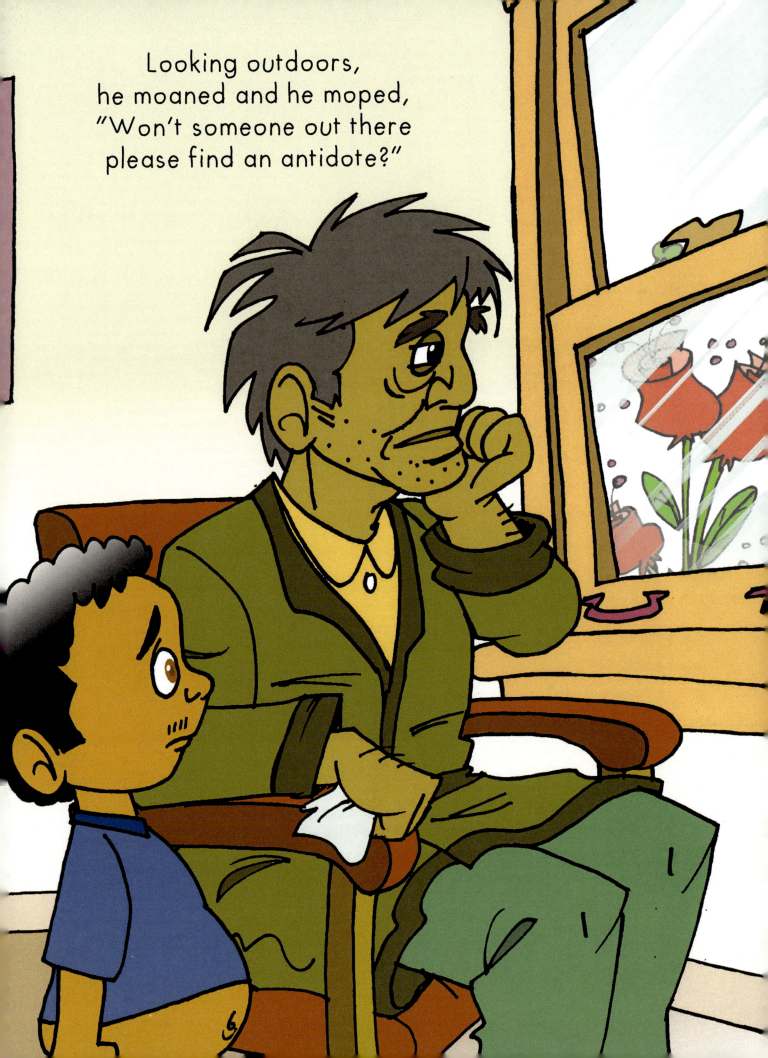
Looking outdoors, he moaned and he moped, "Won't someone out there please find an antidote?"

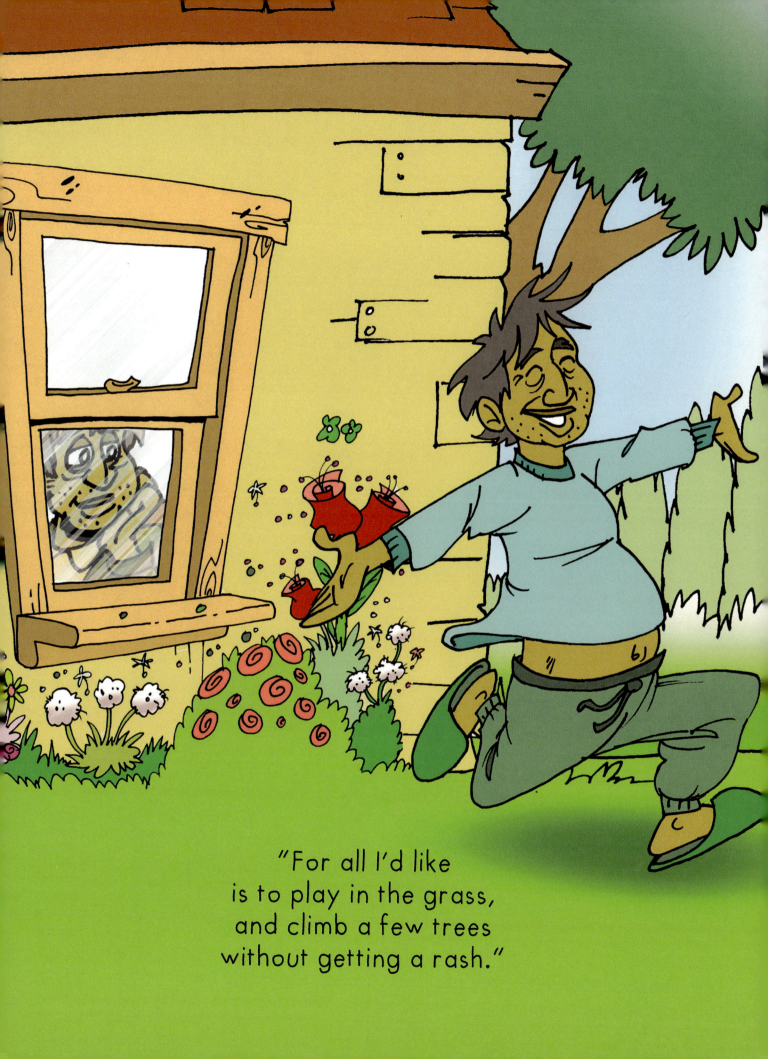

"For all I'd like
is to play in the grass,
and climb a few trees
without getting a rash."

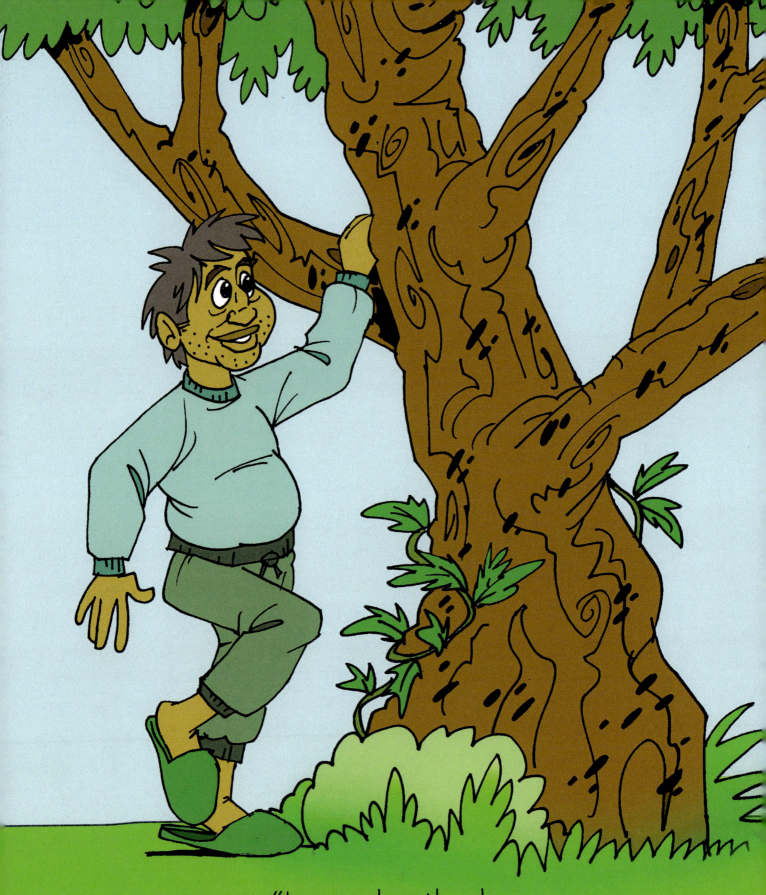

"I remember the days,
I recall them so well.
I remember the sounds,
I remember the smells.

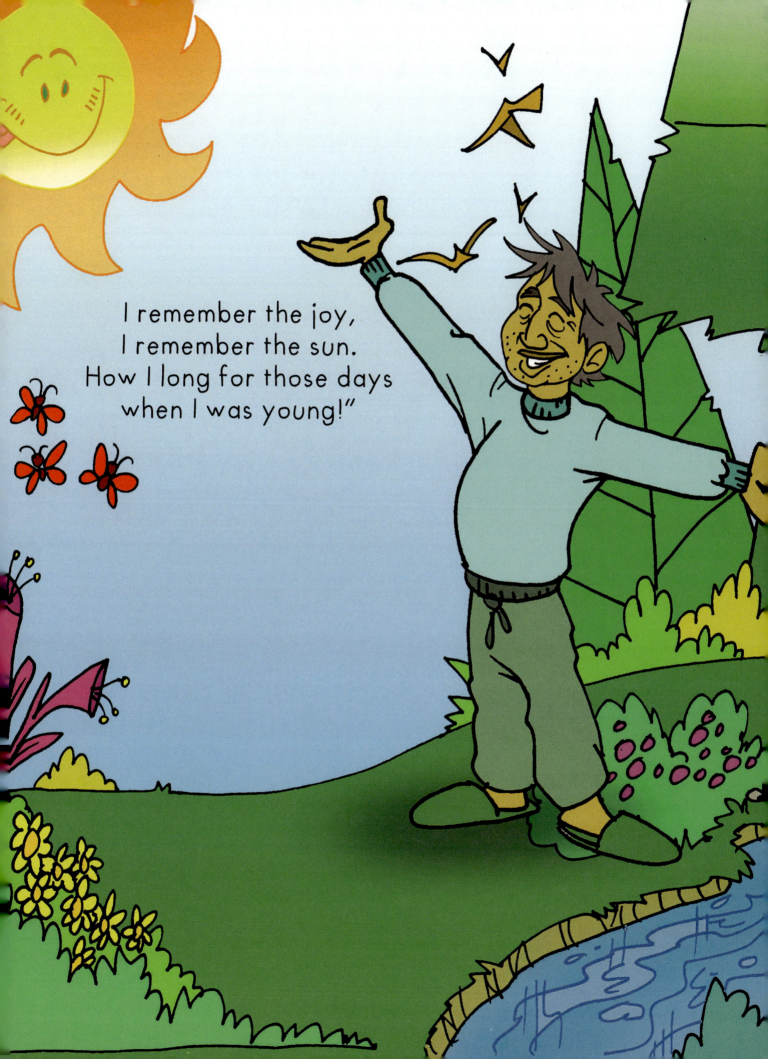

"The sounds of spring
now hurt my head and my brow.
Breathing is tough,
'cause my nose is so stuffed.

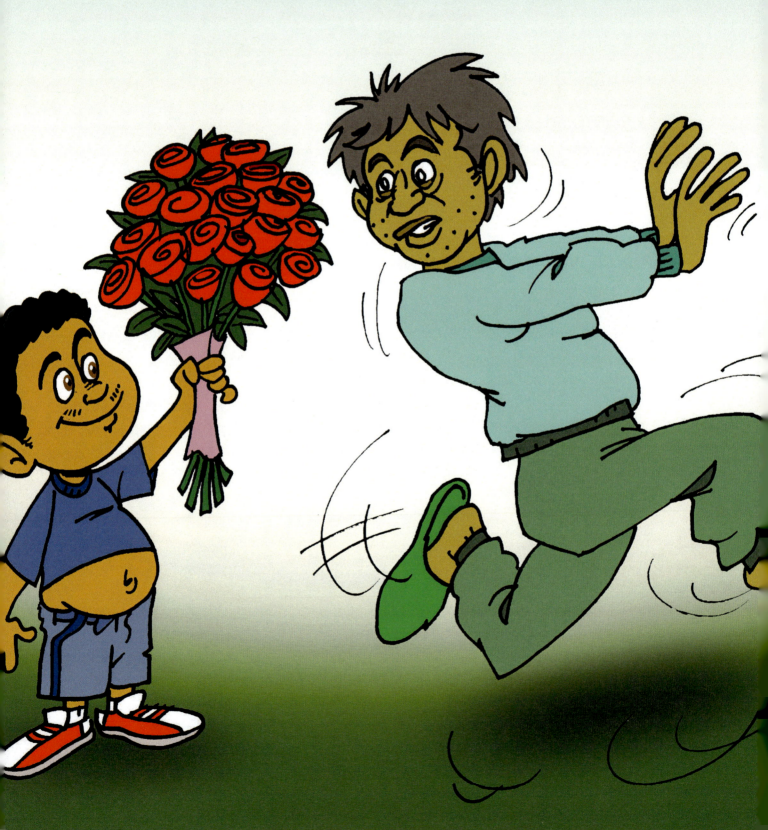

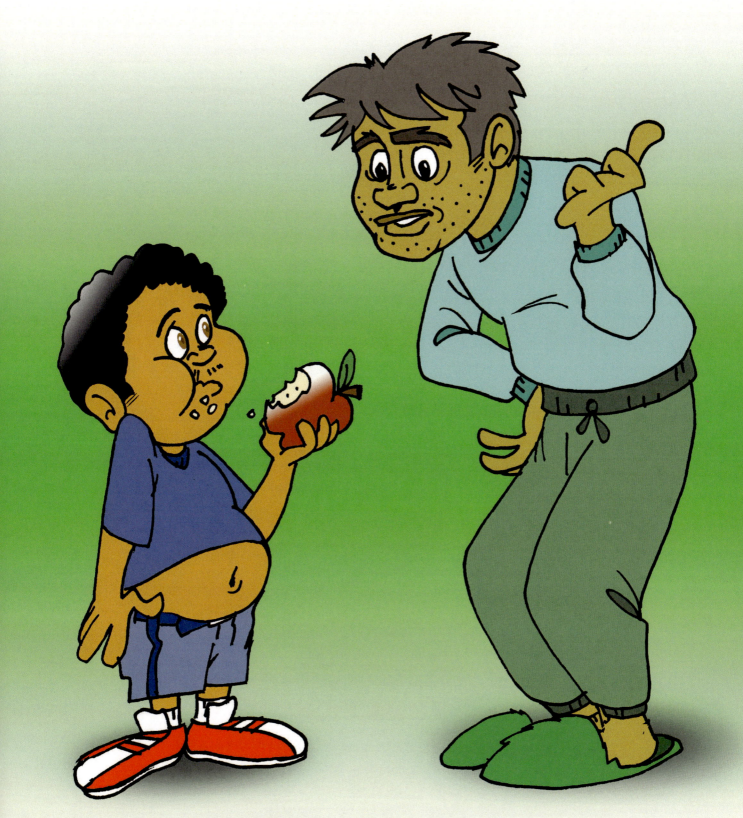

What went wrong
until now, and since then?
What happened at 5?
At 7 and 10?"

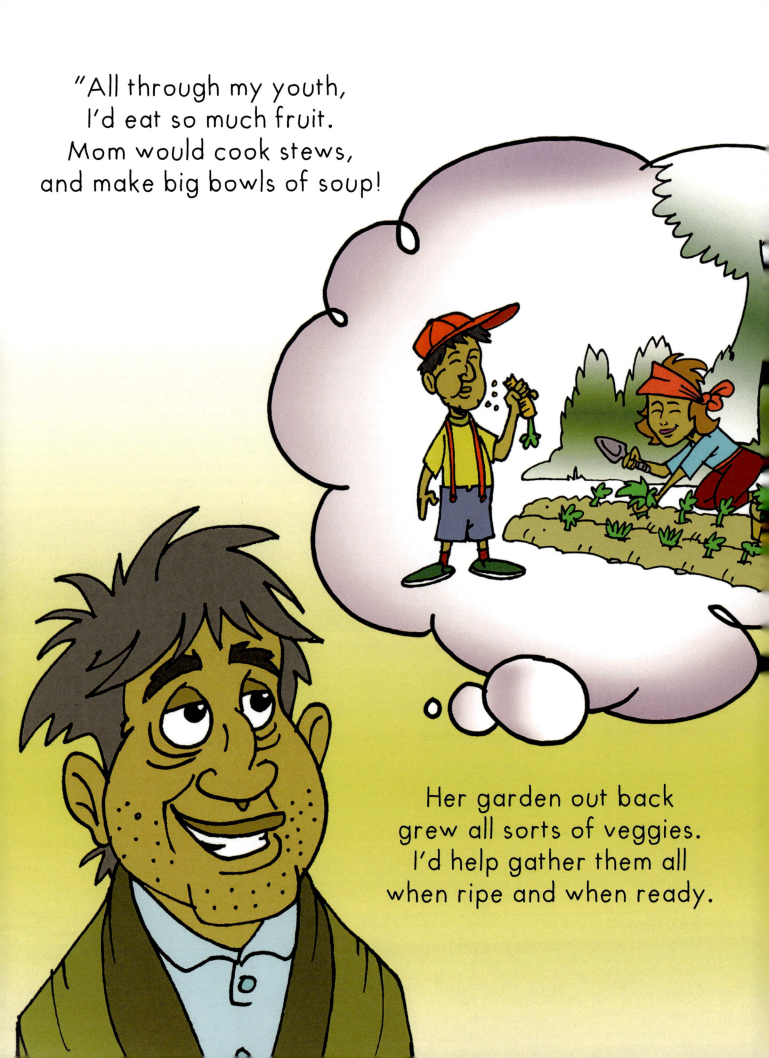

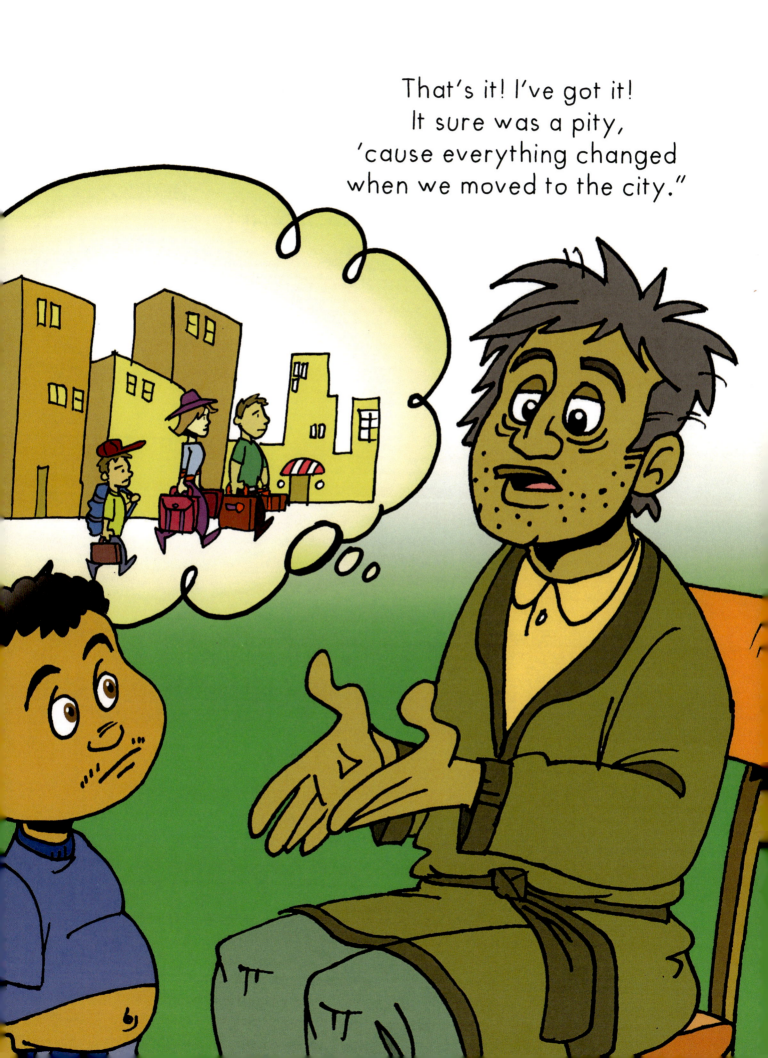

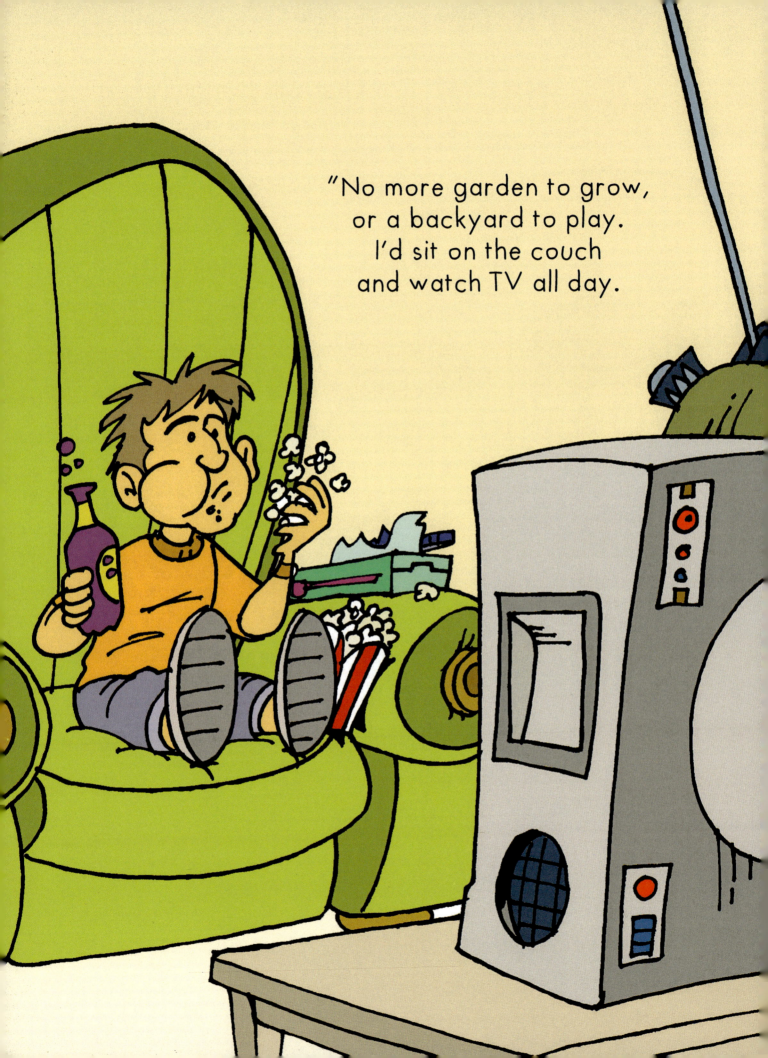

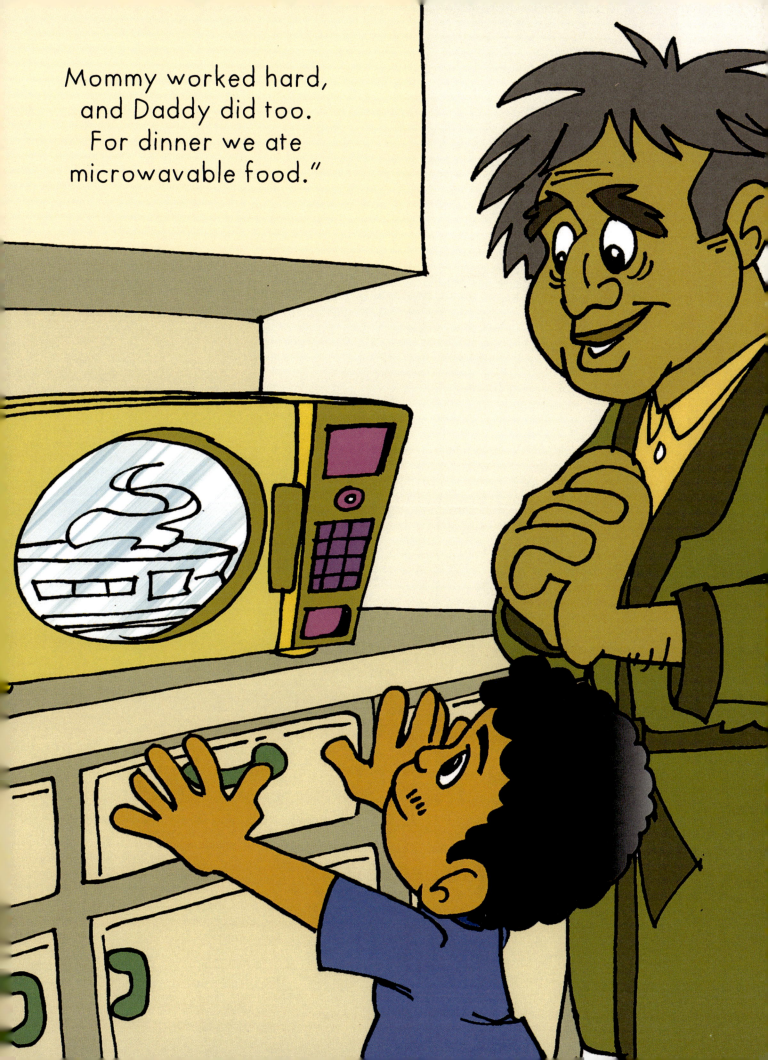

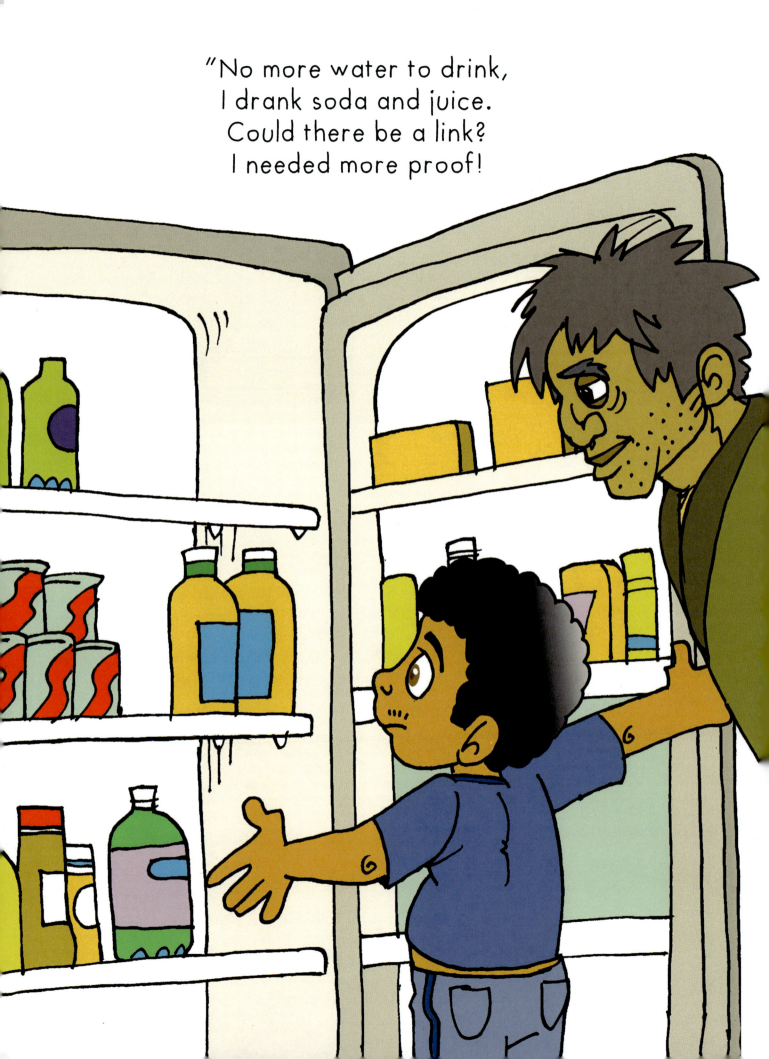
"No more water to drink,
I drank soda and juice.
Could there be a link?
I needed more proof!

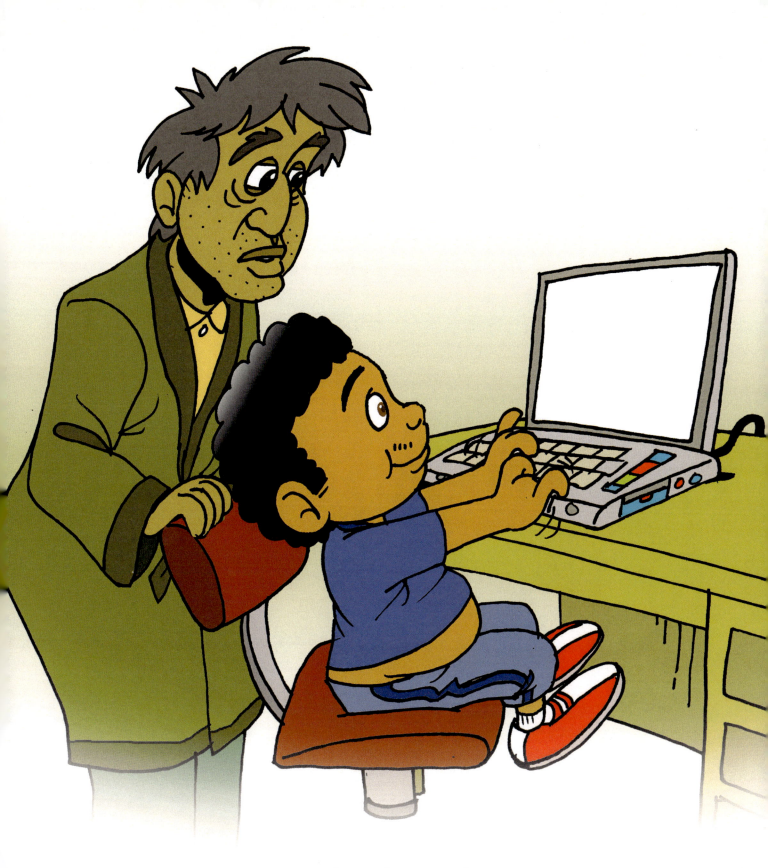

I read and I read,
through books and the net.
About what could come
to my immune system's defense."

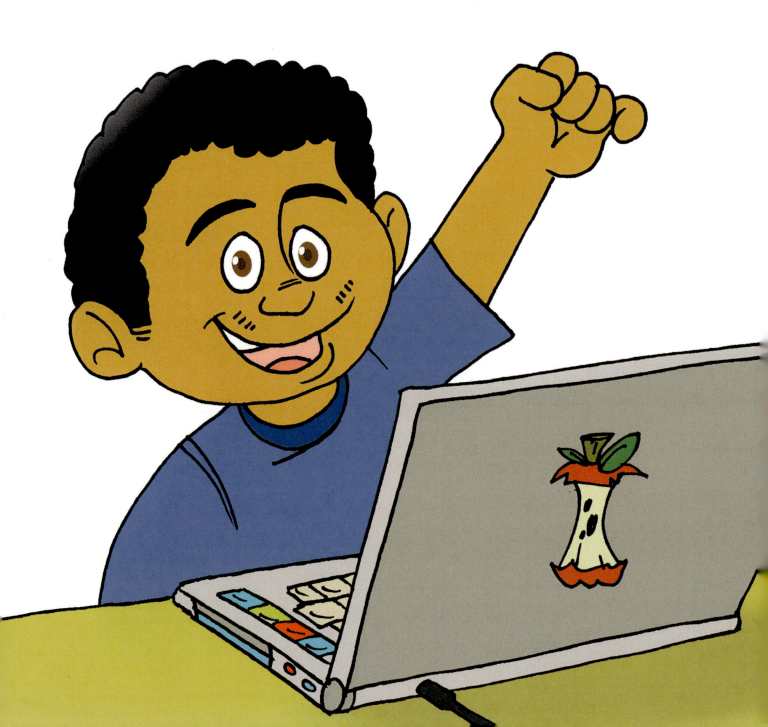

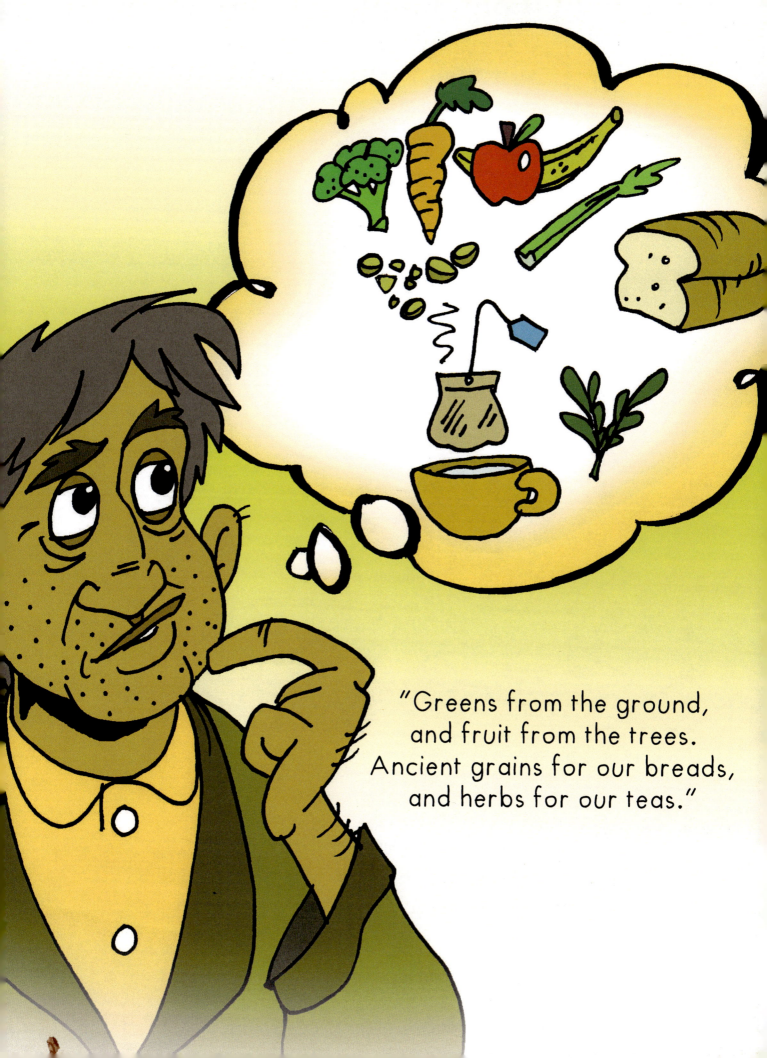

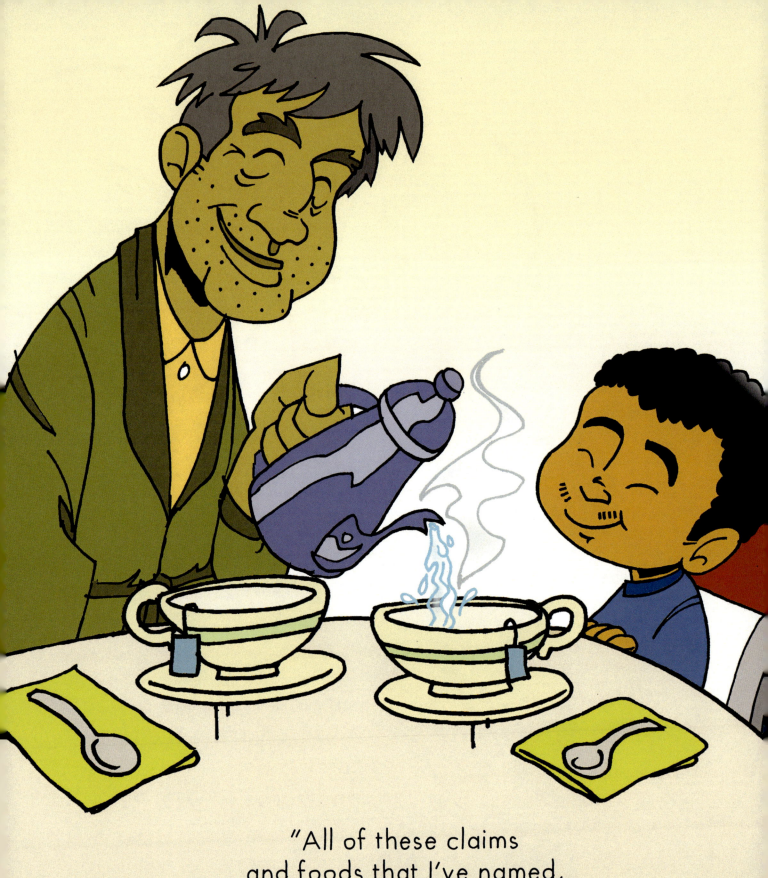

"All of these claims and foods that I've named, fight against keeping our bodies inflamed!

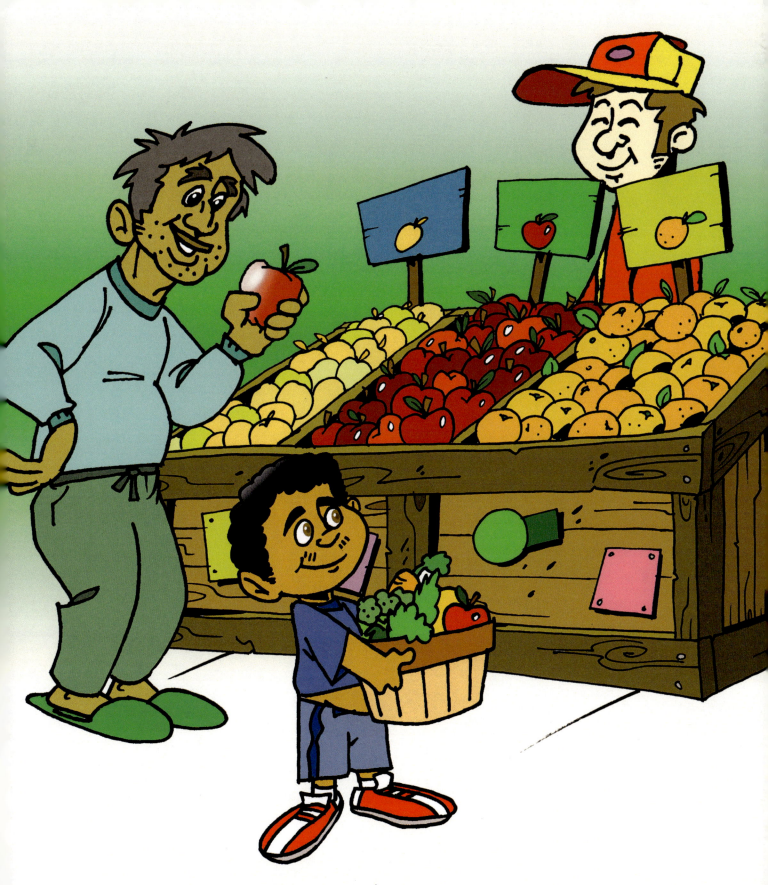

So now that I eat
all natural food,
my allergies are replaced
with a wonderful mood."

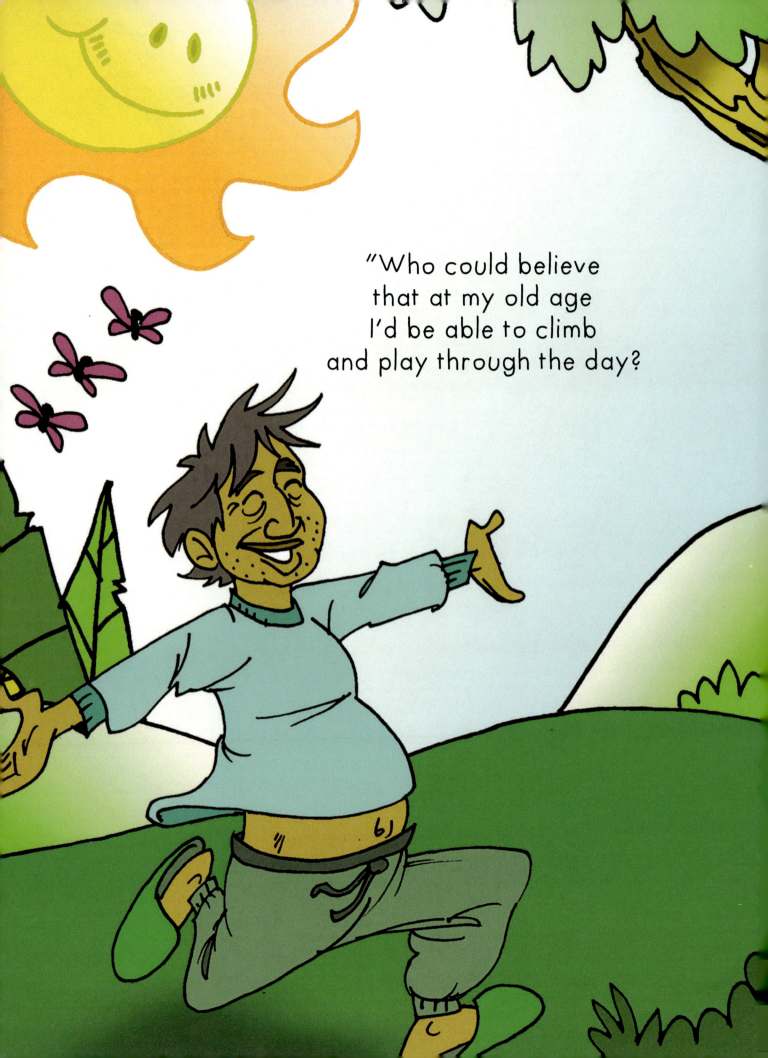

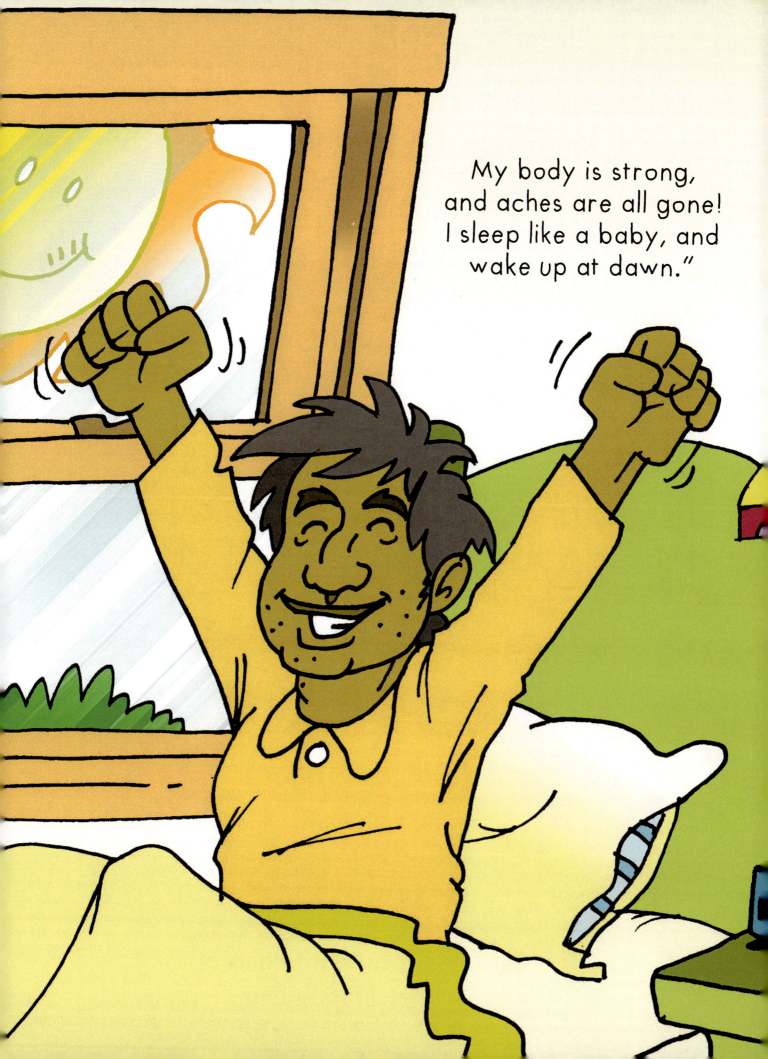

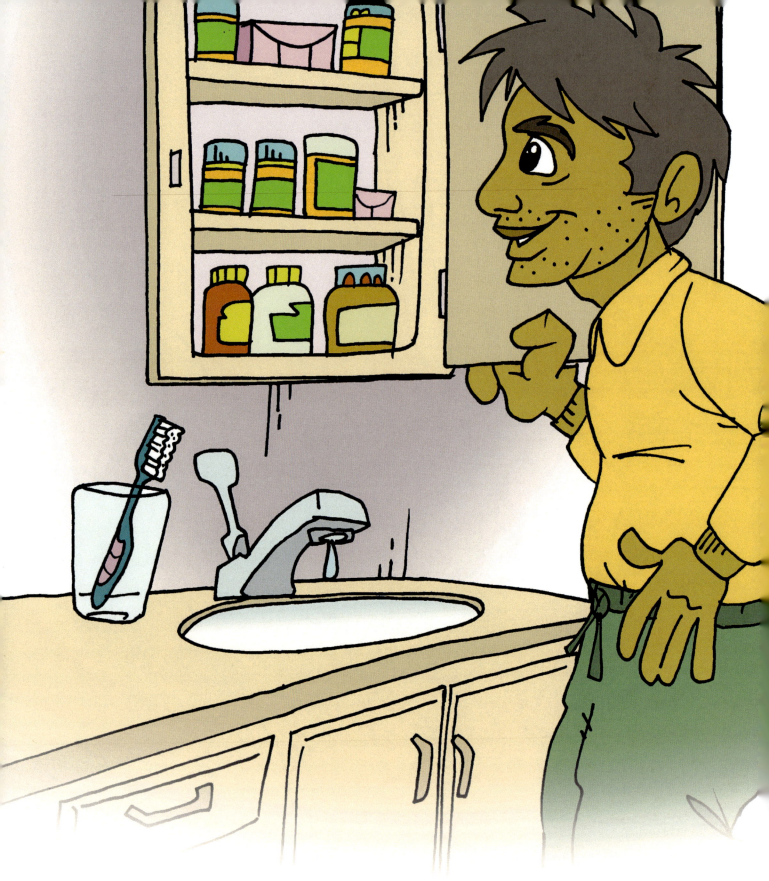

"All of my ills
weren't made better by pills.
But, eating food that is real
has allowed me to heal."

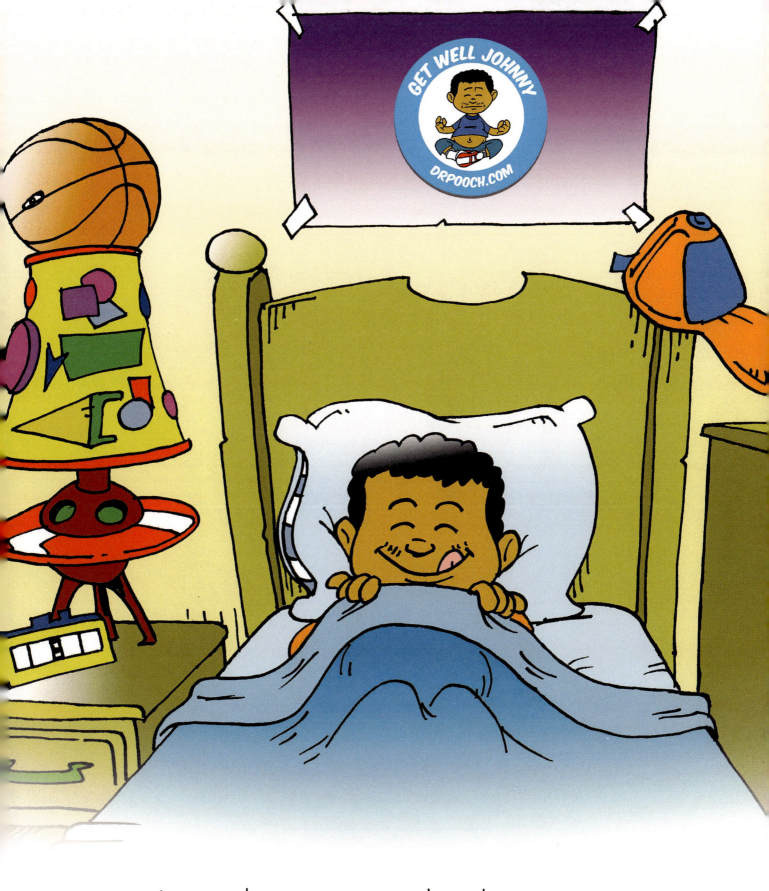

Mustache was amazed at the story
Abuela decided to read him.
And now he's all ready for Allergy Season!

REGGIE REGIMEN'S ALLERGY OCEAN POTION

Hi, my name is Reggie Regimen and together we'll make fun, great tasting raw recipes!

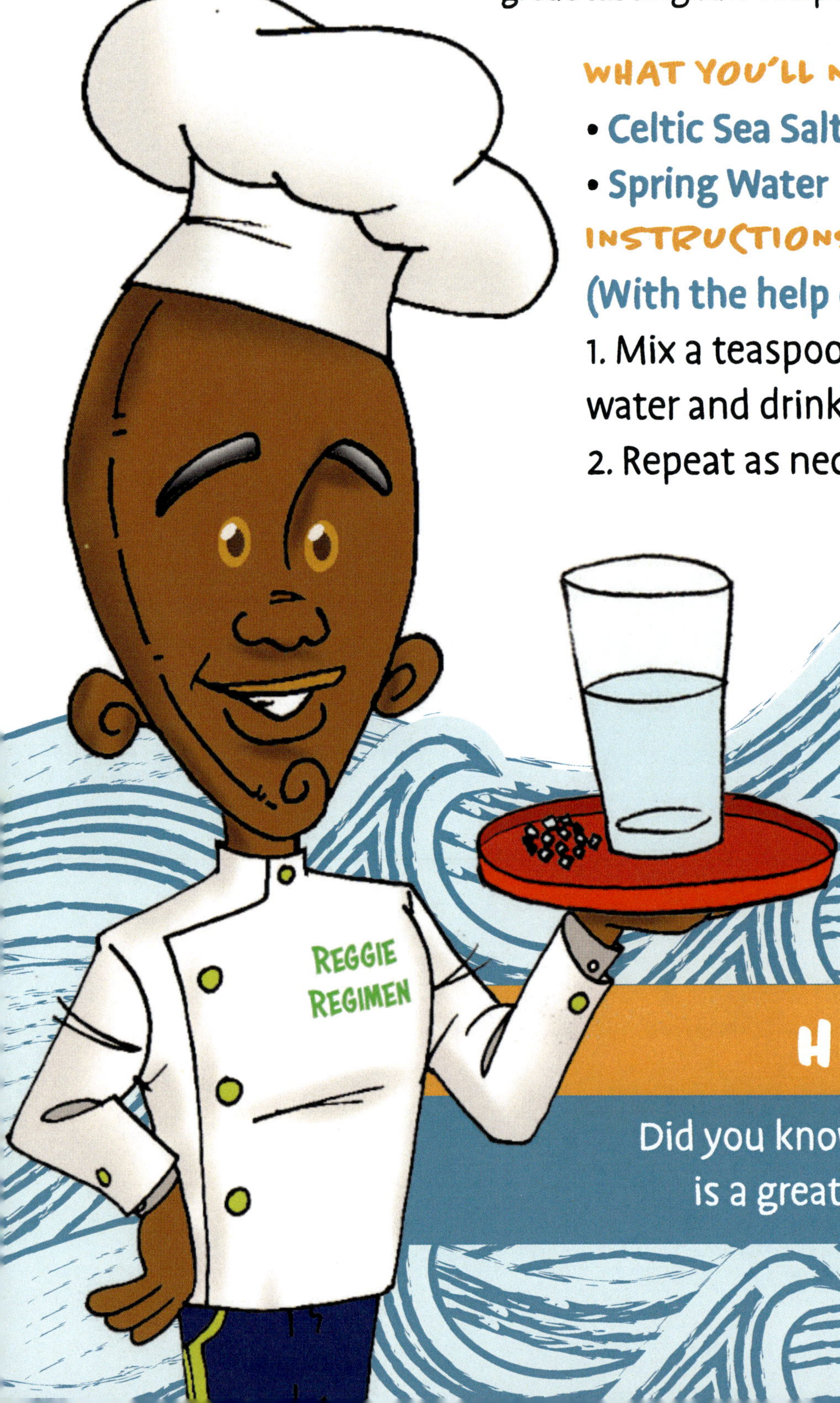

WHAT YOU'LL NEED IS:
- Celtic Sea Salt
- Spring Water

INSTRUCTIONS:
(With the help of an adult)

1. Mix a teaspoon of Celtic Sea Salt with water and drink.
2. Repeat as necessary.

HEALTH TIP

Did you know? Real salt (not table salt) is a great natural antihistamine.

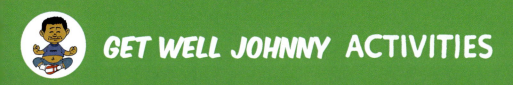

GET WELL JOHNNY ACTIVITIES

LET'S TALK ABOUT
FOOD ALLERGIES

Write the name(s) of any food(s) you or someone you know are allergic to.

_____

_____

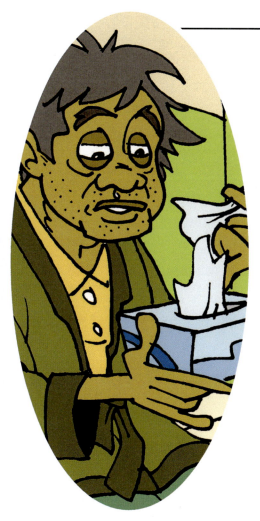

WORD SCRAMBLE
TOP 10 ALLERGIES

1. KIML _____
2. GEGS _____
3. STUN _____
4. TEUNLG _____
5. OYS _____
6. PIRSHM _____
7. LELSHFSIH _____
8. STUNAPE _____
9. HEWAT _____
10. OPLLEN _____

ALLERGIC REACTIONS

Describe an allergic reaction. What happens if someone has an allergic reaction?

_____

_____

KEY — WORD SCRAMBLE: 1. MILK 2. EGGS 3. NUTS 4. GLUTEN 5. SOY 6. SHRIMP 7. SHELLFISH 8. PEANUTS 9. WHEAT 10. POLLEN

LEARN MORE ABOUT NATURAL SUPPLEMENTS

Please prepare & consume under the supervision of an adult!

TURMERIC
This yellow root is a powerful anti-inflammatory food. Coupled with black pepper it becomes even more effective at reducing inflammation!

HONEY
High-quality honeys such as manuka or honey from local farms are great at reducing nasal mucus!

STINGING NETTLES
When allergies pop up in springtime, so do stinging nettles! You will surely find them available online, but who knows, they may be growing like weeds in your own garden!

EYEBRIGHT
Used effectively for centuries, this natural herb is great at relieving red, itchy eyes.

MULLEIN is known to open up the lungs and is another great medicinal herb providing natural relief against allergies!

MINT
Just the wonderful smell of mint could help you breathe better! This wonderful herb can be grown in your very own garden and served as a great healing and nutritious tea!

BAKING SODA
A good quality baking soda is a must have in the pantry when skin rashes or itchy skin occur. Simply make into a paste and apply to affected area for a few minutes!

CASTOR OIL
De-worming practices have been part of our culture for ages. It is only in recent history that we have forgotten this practice. Allergies could be caused by parasitic infection. Natural organic castor oil is a laxative that assists in emptying the stomach and ridding the body of these unwanted guests.

LEARN MORE ABOUT ENVIRONMENTAL FACTORS

Please ask for the help of an adult in approaching any environmental factors or cleaning solutions.

MOLD We could be exposed to mold almost anywhere, both inside and outside of our homes. Reducing the moisture in the air through air conditioners and dehumidifiers can help to create a less friendly environment for mold. Baking soda is a great natural mold cleaner!

DUST MITES These tiny bugs can live in bedding, mattresses, furniture or carpeting! It's hard, if not near impossible, to get rid of dust mites completely. However, natural products such as Diatomaceous Earth can kill them on the spot!

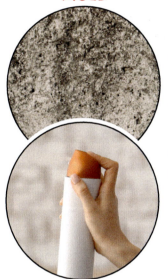

AIR FRESHENER Sprays, scented candles, body washes and perfumes can contain thousands of chemicals that may trigger reactions in many people. Phthalates are a family of chemicals that mimic the effects of hormones in the body. These chemicals are added to fragrances to help smells last longer! Natural herbs such as sage and incense such as frankincense, myrrh, natural oils and soaps are much healthier because they detoxify the air and benefit the body and home in many other ways!

PET DANDER Allergies to pets may occur because their fur is a carrier for an allergen called pet dander, which is composed of tiny flakes of dead skin shed by pets. It is also found in their saliva and even urine. Maintain your animals well! Clean them and feed them natural foods to ensure a shiny healthy coat!

POLLEN are tiny grains from grasses, weeds and trees that travel in the wind. Some plants release their pollen to the air, others use bees to pollenate other flowers. Using herbs and eating anti-inflammatory food may help soothe allergic reactions from the pollen in the air.

TOBACCO Second-hand smoke is very harmful to children and adults. Tobacco is highly sprayed with pesticides and contains more than 7,000 chemicals, more than 70 of which can cause cancer. These chemicals include poisons like formaldehyde, arsenic, DDT and cyanide! Avoid tobacco smoke at all costs!

WEEKLY CHECKLIST ☑

This Activity Sheet Belongs To: _____

✓ **Instructions:** Place a checkmark on each thing you've done each day this week!

This is a weekly checklist kids and/or parents can use to gage where they are in the application of each book's learnings. *Photocopy as needed.*	Sunday	Monday	Tuesday	Wednesday	Thursday	Friday	Saturday
Did I have any trouble breathing today? Breathing is our most basic lifeline.							
Did I eat any green foods today? Greens are great for healthy blood.							
Did I drink any tea today? Nettle, moringa, mint, chamomile, ginger, cloves, cinnamon, cardamom and more make great teas.							
Did I drink at least 3 cups of water? Water is necessary for every function of the body!							
Did I get fresh air today? Sometimes just breathing fresh air makes us feel better!							
Did I poo poo today? #2 is serious business. Chronic constipation can lead to many health problems. Poop everyday!							

HEALTHY CHOICES: Why are healthy habits important? Take notes!

_____

_____

_____

Find fun activities at the end of all Get Well Johnny Books and visit **www.drpooch.com** to learn more!

Allergy Season! Book 5

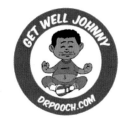

Made in the USA
Middletown, DE
10 March 2022

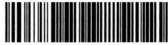